LITTL
VAGINAS

THE LITTLE BOOK OF VAGINAS

An Hachette UK Company
www.hachette.co.uk

Summersdale Publishers Ltd
Part of Octopus Publishing Group Limited
Carmelite House
50 Victoria Embankment
LONDON
EC4Y 0DZ
UK

www.summersdale.com

Printed and bound in Poland

ISBN: 978-1-78783-997-7

The LITTLE BOOK OF VAGINAS

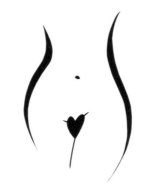

Anna Lou Walker

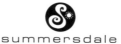

summersdale

For Mum.
Your vagina made it all possible.

Contents

INTRODUCTION

Vagina. Muff. Fanny. Beaver. Pussy. Foof. Coochie. Whatever you call it, the vagina is shrouded in more mystery and taboo than any other body part, despite being owned by around 50 per cent of us. The vulva (all the outer parts of the sex organs), more commonly referred to simply as the "vagina", is sometimes seen as a source of embarrassment and anxiety for people across the globe, but it's also responsible for bringing joy, pleasure and life itself.

It's so important that vagina-owners (after all, not all those with vaginas identify as women) are able to talk about their private parts in all their glory and complexity, both to share their concerns and celebrate their delights with doctors, partners and friends.

In the following pages we will be exploring the vagina, challenging stigmas, busting myths and celebrating what makes our sexual parts so special. In the face of a history that insists upon relegating it to a world of shame, the vagina remains the most powerful and magical of all human organs.

Viva La Vagina!

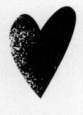

A HISTORY
OF VAGINAS

The vagina has something of a shadowy history. Though worshipped in early cultures as a symbol of nature's power, as organized religion spread across the globe and the concept of shame grew in power and influence, the vagina fell from its pedestal, becoming shrouded in taboo and mystery. In this chapter we'll explore this journey and celebrate the ancient way of looking at the vagina: as the origin of life itself.

WHAT'S IN A NAME?

The etymology of the word "vagina" offers a clue as to why the area has been dismissed as nothing more than a vessel for male pleasure for centuries. In nearly every European language, the word for vagina derives from the Latin *vāgīna*, meaning a "sheath for a sword". Etymologically speaking, the vagina is considered nothing more than a place to store one's, ahem, "weapon".

It's rather surprising, considering its origins, that we readily accept the word "vagina" yet take offence at the use of the swear word "cunt", the derivation of which isn't nearly so offensive. "Cunt" comes from the Old Norse *kunta*, most likely from words meaning "to create" or "woman". Many non-European languages aren't so quick to dismiss the power of the vagina. In Hindi, the word is *yoni*, meaning "source", "fountain" and "nest".

With such reductive European etymology, it's little wonder that a spate of alternative words for vagina has come into common parlance over the years. You're bound to have your favourites but say "vagina" loud and proud and claim back the power over your miraculous sex organ. Taboo who?

THE VAGINA IS AN INSIDE-OUT PENIS

This bizarre myth was believed for thousands of years and still occasionally rears its head today. Leading Roman-era physician Galen instructed his readers to "Think first, please, of the man's [genitals] turned in and extending inward between the rectum and the bladder... the scrotum would take the place of the uteri, with the testes lying outside, next to it on either side."

Essentially, the female reproductive organs were believed to be nothing more than an inverted version of the male's. This, sadly, isn't surprising from a society that believed that men were the superior gender in every way, and women nothing more than imperfect versions of their male counterparts.

In 1994, the US National Institutes of Health decreed that women should be included in clinical trials. Prior to this, very little research was undertaken to discover the ways that the sexes reacted differently to medicine. It was assumed that female and male bodies were essentially doubles, besides the visual discrepancies in their sexual organs.

A (VERY) BRIEF HISTORY

Before the spread of Western theologies, the vagina was often revered. Hindu, Hawaiian, Maori and Irish ancient cultures all feature deities praised for their vaginas, and their powers of fertility and creation.

The history of Western medical research around the vagina, however, can be summed up in just one word: "brief". As the vagina and associated features were believed to simply be an inside-out version of the penis up until the eighteenth century, the discourse remained wildly inaccurate until very recent history. The internal parts of the clitoris, for example, weren't discovered until 1998, thanks to Australian urologist Helen O'Connell.

The cultural limitations placed on women with regards to chastity before marriage and the societal emphasis on sexual "purity" since the Middle Ages have meant that women's sexual health was largely dismissed or ignored up until marriage. As the vagina supposedly only became relevant in its relation to the penis, it was barely considered by men until the point of consummation, and this has impacted heavily on medical fields of research.

MYTHICAL MUFFS

Though our medical history of the vagina is somewhat stunted, a plethora of stories about them can be found throughout ancient history.

In Gaelic mythology, women gathered to "raise their skirts" to defeat Cúchulain, the Irish sun god, in an act known as *anasyrma*. This lifting of the skirts to expose the vagina and harness its power to vanquish enemies recurs several times in history. The ancient Roman philosopher Pliny the Elder described the ways that a menstruating woman could lift her skirts and expose her vagina to end hailstorms, scare pests from crops and calm a storm out at sea.

In nineteenth-century China, old women would line the city walls, exposing their genitals to shock approaching enemies. In 1958, thousands of farming women in Cameroon raised their skirts in protest against new government regulations that would make their lives more difficult.

Then there's Hine-nui-te-po, ruler of the underworld in Maori mythology. An immortal goddess, it is through her vagina that her enemies attempted to vanquish her, but Hine-nui-te-po defeated them each time by casually crushing them between her powerful thighs.

VAGINA VALLEY

Created around 35,000 BC, the crude vagina carved into the rockface of a cave in Vézère Valley, France is the first known artistic depiction of the sex organ. Discovered in 1994, the engraving is a simple circle with a line struck from the middle point downward. Similar depictions have been found in other Stone Age sites carved from mammoth molars, bones or limestone, also showcasing the simple circle and line design.

Researchers were very excited by the discovery, because it could be considered the earliest example of humanity's relationship with our sexuality. It may even mark the point at which intercourse changed from a necessary biological function to an activity engaged in for pleasure.

Not only is this the earliest known depiction of a vagina, but it's also the world's oldest cave engraving full stop. How appropriate that the first known carved expressions of human art would be depicting the origin of all human life itself.

PUNANI POETRY

Around 3000 BC, Sumerian society (in modern-day Iraq) paid worship to a goddess named Ishtar, regarded as divine due to the wetness of her vagina. Cardi B and Megan Thee Stallion would be proud.

According to poetic texts from the time, Ishtar sang the following to her mortal lover, a shepherd king named Dumuzi: "Who will plough my high field? Who will plough my wet ground? As for me, the young woman, who will plough my vulva? Who will station the ox there?"

Hearing her poetic cry, her lover soon shouted back, "I, Dumuzi the King, will plough your vulva".

Delighted, Ishtar called back, "Then plough my vulva, man of my heart!"

The two made love, and when Dumuzi ejaculated, plants were seeded and began to grow all around the lovers. In Sumerian society, the vagina and penis were considered equal partners in the role of fertilization of the land and regeneration of the people.

IT CAN ACHE FOR US AND STRETCH FOR US, DIE FOR US AND BLEED AND BLEED US INTO THIS DIFFICULT, WONDROUS WORLD.

Eve Ensler

TEMPLE OF POON

Long before vaginas became taboo, they were not only openly worshipped and deified, but temples were built in their honour.

In the ancient Greek city of Priene, a temple was built in the fifth century BC and decorated with adornments celebrating a goddess less known to modern audiences than her contemporaries Aphrodite, Hera or Athena.

That deity is Baubo, and each statue of her within the temple walls represents her in the same way – a beautiful woman's face with elaborate hair sitting directly atop a pair of voluptuous legs. Instead of a chin, she has a vagina, the hint of a smile playing across her face. Baubo was the goddess of mirth, a sexually liberated figure who enjoyed bawdy humour, and was known to make her fellow goddesses laugh with a flash of her vagina.

Thousands made pilgrimages to honour Baubo's role in Greek legend, to join festivities in which they would re-enact the stories of their gods. Among the celebrations was a ceremonial lifting of the skirts, to honour Baubo's own penchant for flashing.

Baubo's role was to remind devotees of the regenerative power of the vagina, and her origins can be traced back even further than ancient Greece. In ancient Phoenicia she was known as Baev and worshipped as the "guardian of the source". In ancient Egypt she was Bebt, and popular mass-produced statues of the goddess showed her defiantly flashing her vagina.

Baubo's story resonated deeply in these patriarchal societies, perhaps offering women a moment of recognition for the bonds they quietly shared, and for the transformative power of laughter to unite them in the face of oppression.

Around AD 200, as Christians began to convert the Greeks, the worships of old were mocked, and the vagina was reconceptualized as sinful and shameful. As such, Baubo fell out of favour in popular culture, though she does make occasional reappearances. In Johann Wolfgang von Goethe's nineteenth-century play *Faust*, she is portrayed as an occult, witch-like figure. She also appears in the writing of philosopher Friedrich Nietzsche and psychologist Sigmund Freud.

A RARE JEWEL

According to ancient Hindu mythology, the vagina – or *yoni* as it's known in Hindi – is to be revered as the source of all existence. The symbol of this great power dates back to 4000 BC in the form of the goddess Shakti. According to Hindu tradition, Shakti has the power to birth, sustain, and to destroy – she is the master of all creative energies. One of the oldest depictions of Shakti in India is the simple form of a triangle, representing the vagina.

Shaktism, a major sect of Hinduism, focuses worship on Shakti as the representation of the femininity of the Supreme Divine. The *Shakti Sangama Tantra* states "Woman is the creator of the universe, the universe is her form; woman is the foundation of the world, she is the true form of the body. In woman is the form of all things, of all that lives and moves in the world. There is no jewel rarer than woman, no condition superior to that of a woman."

THE KAMA SUTRA

Though all too often reduced to glossy sex tip spreads in magazines that stray far from the truth of the original texts, the Kama Sutra is an ancient Sanskrit guide to sexual and personal fulfilment written around 400 BC. It describes ways to find pleasure and happiness in both hetero and gay and lesbian relationships, with a variety of techniques for foreplay, sex, flirtation and choosing the perfect partner.

The vagina, or *yoni*, is described in the Kama Sutra as belonging to one of three categories: "female deer", "mares" or "female elephants", depending on its depth. It is suggested that they match with penises, or *lingams*, of equal size, depicted as the "hare man", the "bull man" and the "stallion man".

This quote from the *Brihadaranyaka Upanishad* is said to be one of the inspiring foundational texts of the Kama Sutra: "A fire – that is what a woman is... Her firewood is the vulva, her smoke is the pubic hair, her flame is the vagina, when one penetrates her, that is her embers, and her sparks are the climax."

LATIN LUST

The Romans didn't have the celebratory view of vaginas that many other ancient cultures enjoyed. Instead, Latin texts usually point to the vagina as the origin of sin – a dangerous, powerful source to be controlled by the man.

One such story is that of Messalina, wife to the Emperor Claudius, who reigned AD 41–45. Following her death, legends concerning her alleged promiscuity began to circulate. In his *Satires*, the Roman poet Juvenal describes how the young empress abandoned the palace at night in order to satiate her endless sexual urges. Messalina would head to a nearby brothel, where she would take lover after lover, returning to the palace only once the brothel closed, with her "taut sex still burning".

Frustrated by the inability to satisfy her raging lust, Messalina embarked on more and more extreme sexual escapades, challenging a prostitute to a 24-hour sex-a-thon, in which she enjoyed 25 different partners. According to the legend, Claudius tired of his wife's sexual dominance, and ordered her execution – the only way he could think to end her sexual deviance.

BEAVERS BITE BACK

Fear of the *vagina dentata* – or toothed vagina – existed long before the 2007 comedy horror *Teeth* hit cinemas. In this world view, the vagina is a toothed and hungry beast, and copulation something of an epic battle to fertilization, with the willing hero tasked with defanging the vagina before he can enjoy her and sow his seed. The ancient Greek word for semen, *sema*, translated as "food", while the Bavarian German word for vagina *fotze*, literally translates as "mouth".

In the Amazonian Yanomami tribe, the words for sex and eating are the same, and the word for "pregnant" translates as "fully fed". Meanwhile, in Brazil, the Mundurucu tribe call the vagina the "crocodile's mouth".

In some parts of the world, this toothy mythology has been given real-world uses. South African inventor Sonnet Ehlers created an anti-rape device known as RapeX, essentially a female condom lined with painful barbs that can only be removed from the attacker's penis through surgery.

SHEELA NA GIGS

Wander around a Norman church in parts of Europe and you might be surprised by a rather unusual carving perched among the traditional gargoyles and saints. Sheela Na Gigs, which were created in France and Spain in the eleventh century AD before appearing in the UK and Ireland in the twelfth century, are cartoon-like statues of nude women, spreading wide their crudely carved labia to present their vagina to the surprised viewer.

Speaking about their presence on so many places of worship, a spokesman for the Church of England said, "As with other gargoyles and grotesques, it is sometimes surprising to modern eyes to encounter them in a religious context. But they reflect the diversity of architectural ornament found on churches up and down the country."

Historians disagree about the purpose of these statues. While some believe they were intended to ward off evil spirits, others believe their placement on churches alludes to the early Christian views of female lust and sexuality as inherently sinful. Others suggest that they are a nod to pre-Christian, pagan mother-goddess worship.

Young brides were sometimes required to look at and touch Sheela Na Gig figures before their wedding day, suggesting that they either served as a fertility amulet, or as a deterrent for sexually deviant behaviour within the marriage. The crude, almost scary nature of their appearance has also been seen as a sign that they were made to depict "crones", scaring women away from lustful behaviour with the sight of what they could become.

American midwife and author Ina May Gaskin suggests a different theory entirely. In her book *Ina May's Guide to Childbirth*, she shares her belief that these figures were actually intended to "reassure young women about the capabilities of their bodies in birth". Indeed, Gaskin muses that she'd rather like renditions of Sheela Na Gigs to decorate the birthing rooms of our modern maternity units.

VICTORIAN VAGINAS

We generally think of the Victorian era as stifling years for vagina-owners. "The majority of women," one doctor wrote, "(happily for them), are not troubled with sexual feelings of any kind." After all, this was the period where chastity was prized above all else in a woman, and ladies could barely entertain a prospective spouse without the aid of a chaperone. But all was perhaps not as it seems.

In the 1890s, Dr Clelia Duel Mosher – an American physician and woman's health advocate who frowned upon the ruling stereotypes around women's sexuality of the day – started a 20-year survey on the sexual habits and preferences of Victorian women.

Though never published in her lifetime, the survey of 45 women is extremely revealing as to the interior sexual world of Victorian vagina-owners. With regard to orgasms, one respondent described the "nerve-wracking", "unbalancing" effect of a long spell of sex without orgasm, while another claimed that men had "not been properly trained" in pleasuring women.

WARTIME WOES

The First and Second World Wars led to a significant shift in the ways women's sexual freedoms were considered.

With husbands and fathers away fighting on foreign soil, women rose to become the heads of their households, with more autonomy and freedom over their everyday lives than they had ever enjoyed before. Many also came into employment for the first time in their lives, working as nurses or in artillery factories, often taking over jobs previously held by their husbands, which offered them a new financial freedom too.

Some historians have argued that this period also gave rise to an increase in promiscuity. The opportunities for sexual encounters were certainly greater, and records show a rise in births to single mothers during the Second World War. Women were far more visible in society and thrown into the paths of prospective partners more often, particularly those women who undertook positions such as train conductors or working in hospitality, where they'd meet men from out of town.

Notions around women's sexualities were changing, as were the limits of the oppressions women were willing to endure in the name of chastity.

A WARTIME "SOLUTION"

The rates of sexually transmitted diseases among soldiers led to great fear from governments of the "threat" of sexually available women. In the US, dramatic measures were taken. From the First World War through to the

1950s, sexually active women were rounded up and quarantined as part of "The American Plan" to protect soldiers. Stays at these detention centres often involved invasive medical inspections and painful "treatments", including the application of arsenic, mercury and bismuth to visible areas of infection, including genitals.

It was assumed, in line with the gender politics of the time, that men were not the carriers of disease; rather, they were victims of infected women. Historian Karin L. Zipf notes that these "gender and class-based anti-prostitution and venereal disease control laws... reinforced a double standard, one that acknowledged the sexual impulses of men while it repressively punished women."

One social hygienist at the time went so far as to say, "It is generally recognized that a bad and diseased woman can do more harm than any German fleet of airplanes." The last centres set up to "solve" this "girl problem" weren't closed until 1953.

THE SWINGING SIXTIES

The 1960s revolutionized women's sexual freedom with the introduction of the contraceptive pill. Abortion was still illegal in both the US and the UK and the pill removed the very real threat of unwanted pregnancy. Abortion was not legalized until 1968 in the UK, and 1973 in the US. By 1965, six million American women were taking the pill. Women had never before had such control over their sex life and it prioritized the pursuit of pleasure like never before – so much so that this era is now referred to as the "sexual revolution".

For the first time, sex outside of marriage was becoming socially acceptable. The proportion of women in the US who delayed sexual intercourse until marriage declined from 48 per cent in 1960 to 21 per cent in 1975. The number of births to unmarried women also increased from 5 per cent in 1960 to 19 per cent in 1982.

> The sixties also heralded an outpouring of feminist writing and protest, including Betty Friedan's hugely significant book, *The Feminine Mystique*, which challenged people's conceptions of female sexuality and agency, articulating for the first time in print the problems shared by women across the globe.

BEATING AROUND THE BUSH

Believe it or not, the trend for a hairless vagina was doing the rounds long before widespread access to pornography or the infamous "Brazilian" episode of *Sex and the City* ("you can't hide your light under a bush"). Ancient Egyptians removed all of their body hair using sharp flints or pumice stones, as did women in many Middle Eastern cultures and in ancient Turkey. In ancient Greece, meanwhile, appearing at the public baths with visible pubic hair would have been scandalous. Instead, a smooth pubic mound was achieved through individual plucking of each hair – suddenly a wax doesn't sound so painful.

In medieval Europe, the trend was largely to allow pubic hair to grow as wild and free as nature intended it, though a few women did experiment with home-made hair-removal cream. This was also the time of the first pubic wig, aka a merkin, which was first documented in 1450. And the trend wasn't going anywhere – in 1714, author Alexander Smith wrote with delight about "the hairy circle of a prostitute's merkin."

The bush reigned supreme until the early twentieth century. The shortage of nylon during the war meant that disposable razors were a far more common fixture in women's bathrooms, as they could no longer conceal hairy pins under a pair of tights. It wasn't too far a stretch to think of the other ways these new tools could be utilized.

Pubic hair came back in a big and bushy way in the sixties and seventies, however, when "free love" and second-wave feminism were in full swing. It was only trumped with the dawn of the 1990s, when the full Hollywood wax became a celebrity trend. So common did the style become that by 2013 doctors declared that pubic lice (also known as crabs) had become an endangered species.

When it comes to pubic styling, free choice is the order of the day. Like a little fluff on your foof? Work it. Prefer things smooth? Do your thing. Experiment all you like, but only settle on the look that makes you feel the most comfortable and confident. After all, it's nobody's vagina but yours.

FOR ME, THE VAGINA IS SUCH AN INTEGRAL PART OF THE BODY. WE THINK THE VAGINA IS ON THE OUTSIDE. I SAY GRAB A MIRROR AND PLAY ALONG. GET IN THERE. LEARN ABOUT IT.

Cameron Diaz

THE VAGINA REVOLUTION

In 1970, the first Women's Liberation Conference was held in England, and in the same year, Australian activist Germaine Greer published her influential book, *The Female Eunuch*. In it, she argued that traditional gender roles were repressing women's sexuality and that women needed to rediscover their vaginas. "If you think you are emancipated," she wrote, "you might consider the idea of tasting your own menstrual blood. If it makes you sick, you've got a long way to go, baby."

The revolution of the seventies extended into the eighties, spanning all forms of culture. In fashion designer Vivienne Westwood's collection *Voyage to Cythera*, models walked the catwalk in strategically placed fig leaves.

The message behind the show, and the controversy it provoked, were debated by critics. But one thing was for certain – it thrust the vagina into the spotlight as a point of conversation for the masses. "When I first did the fig leaf in 1989," Westwood said later, "I just kept screaming. It was so porno and so hilariously mad. Then I got used to it, and I think it looks so elegant and ironic."

VAGINAS IN MODERN PROTEST

During the Black Lives Matter protests of 2020 following the murder of George Floyd at the hands of the Minneapolis Police Department, an unidentified protestor in Portland, Oregon, earned the nickname "Naked Athena" after removing her clothes, sitting on the tarmac and opening her legs, placing herself between police and protestors. She didn't say a word. One policeman shot her in the foot with a rubber ball. She calmly raised it to show him the blood.

"None of these [protestors] have weapons," she explained on the podcast *Unrefined Sophisticates*. "Empty their pockets, take off their clothes – nobody has weapons here. I just wanted them [the police] to see what they're shooting at... There was a very deep feminine place in myself that felt provoked... This fury arose in me... I said, 'I want to be naked. I want to confront them.'"

Officers left just 10 minutes after the Naked Athena's display.

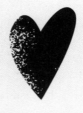

ANATOMY OF THE VAGINA

An incredible 65 per cent of women in Western countries are uncomfortable with the word "vagina" and 45 per cent say they never talk about their vaginal health with anyone, including their doctor. This chapter will work through each part of the vulva, from the outer lips in to the uterus, and introduce you to the beautiful complexity of the vagina, without the shame.

VAGINAS SMELL LIKE FISH

Self-consciousness around smell is something most vagina-owners experience at some point. Indeed, there are a host of products on the market designed to neutralize the vaginal "odour". Gwyneth Paltrow hit headlines in 2019 for a rather unusual addition to her wellness store, Goop: a candle named "This Smells Like My Vagina" with notes of geranium, citrus and rose.

Contrary to the fishy myth and the vagina-scenting industry that has popped up around it, healthy vaginas simply smell of… well… vagina. Each has its own unique scent, and only you can know what "normal" means for you. Many describe their smell as musky, tangy, coppery or even reminiscent of beer. Indeed, the healthy bacteria that dominate vaginas – known as *lactobacilli* – can also be found in yoghurt, sourdough bread and some beers, which is why the scents have common ground.

If your vagina *does* smell like fish, it's most likely the sign of a common infection such as bacterial vaginosis (see page 132), which can be cleared up easily with a trip to your doctor.

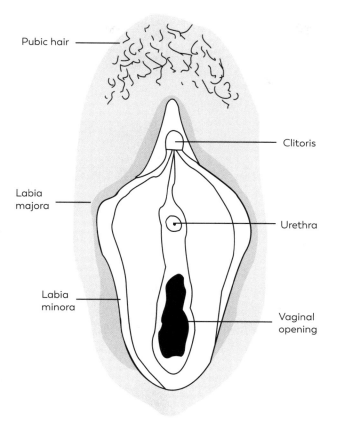

Pubic hair

Clitoris

Labia
majora

Urethra

Labia
minora

Vaginal
opening

PUBIC HAIR

Type "pubic hair" into a search engine and the suggested queries are extremely revealing: "pubic hair removal cream", "pubic hair trimmer", "pubic hair dye". While changing the appearance of your bush can be fun – experimenting with shapes, lengths and colours – it's easy to forget the clever role your down-there hair plays in looking after your vaginal health.

The skin surrounding your vagina is extremely sensitive, and one of the main benefits of rocking your pubic hair *au naturel* is that it provides a fluffy cushion against harsh friction during sex, preventing painful chafing to your nether regions – ouch!

Pubic hair also stops harmful bacteria from entering the body by trapping dirt, sweat and micro-organisms before they can reach the vagina. According to research from 2017, pubic hair may even play a role in reducing the risk of contracting sexually transmitted diseases.

Scientists have suggested that pubic hair aids the transmission of pheromones, increasing how attractive we will appear to prospective romantic interests. Winner!

THE LABIA

The labia majora are the first thing you'll see when looking at your vagina. They are the two fatty folds of skin that join to form a slit and protect the sensitive parts of your vagina from the outside world.

The words "labia majora" come from the Latin for "big lips". The labia majora have two sides. The dry outside is a similar skin to that which covers the rest of the body and is covered in pubic hair growth, while the hairless inside is smooth, usually a darker or browner/pinker colour, and needs to remain slightly moist for optimal vaginal comfort.

Gently part your labia majora and you'll be met with the labia minora. These smaller lips start with a top fold that forms the cosy hood of the clitoris and extend downward toward the vagina. The minora are made from much thinner skin than the majora and are lined with a mucous membrane, with a surface kept moist through the secretion of fluid by their specialized cells.

The appearance of the labia minora varies wildly from person to person. While for some they protrude outside of the labia majora, for others they are tucked away and not visible without parting the outer lips. For some, the labia minora are unsymmetrical, and for others they are exactly even.

Across the world, the idea of what makes the labia minora "ideal" varies wildly. In Europe and the US, labiaplasty (a surgery that reduces the size of the labia minora) has seen a huge increase in recent years, in tandem with the rise of pornography consumption. In Rwanda, however, large lips are considered the most attractive and in Japan, uneven labia minora are seen as extremely desirable and known as the "winged butterfly". To see just how diverse the appearance of the labia minora can be, visit www.greatwallofvagina. co.uk/great-wall-vagina-panels to explore a sculpture created by artist Jamie McCartney, formed from the casts of 400 different vulvas.

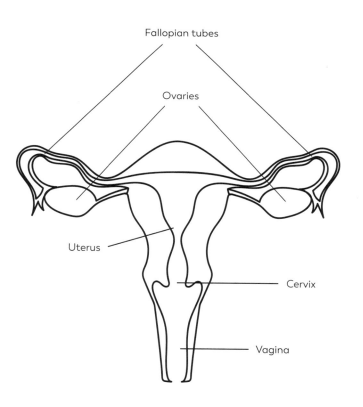

Fallopian tubes

Ovaries

Uterus

Cervix

Vagina

THE CLITORIS

The clitoris you can see is just the tip of the iceberg when it comes to your pleasure organ, though incredibly we only discovered this in 1998, thanks to the Australian urologist Helen O'Connell.

The visible part of the clitoris, which sits under the fold of the labia minora known as the "clitoral hood" and looks rather like a pink pea, is known as the "glans". It is the primary source of sexual pleasure for vagina-owners, and most who are able to reach orgasm do so through its stimulation.

The full, internal clitoris organ looks rather like a wishbone, extending down either side of the vagina. The glans itself is home to around 8,000 sensory nerve endings, twice as many as the penis, and it is the only organ in the human body whose sole purpose is to provide pleasure. At the moment of orgasm, the clitoris spreads that amazing sensation to 15,000 other nerves in the pelvic region, which is why the big O can feel so all-consuming.

The clitoris can be stimulated in a variety of ways, including gently stroking with fingers, oral stimulation with the lips and tongue or through the friction of rubbing the area against something else. However it is being pleasured, lubrication almost always heightens the experience.

Some may notice that as the blood rushes to their clitoris with arousal, it becomes engorged, while for others the clitoral size will barely change. Sensitivity of the clitoris also varies from person to person. For some, the glans is so sensitive that direct contact can be uncomfortable, and pleasure is best provided through stimulation of the surrounding area.

You've probably heard of the G-spot before, but you might be surprised to know that this is actually still the clitoris, just stimulated internally. For some people, this area isn't sensitive enough to notice, while for others, it's the key to orgasm. This may explain why some can orgasm through penetrative sex, while others require external stimulation to reach their moment of bliss.

THE URETHRA

The urethra is the small opening above the vagina through which you urinate. Its job is to transport urine from the bladder and out of your body. The lining of the urethra is made up of a layer of cells known as the epithelium, which produce mucus to protect the urethra from the corrosive elements of urine.

Due to its proximity to the vagina, there is a higher risk of vagina-owners contracting urinary tract infections (UTIs) than people with a penis. UTIs such as cystitis make the sufferer feel an increased need to urinate, and a burning sensation when they pee. There may also be blood in the urine or pain in the lower tummy. The experience can be extremely uncomfortable and sometimes painful.

To avoid contracting UTIs, it's advisable to wipe front to back when using the toilet and to always urinate after penetrative sex, which expels damaging bacteria from the urethra before it can do damage.

THE VAGINA

The vagina is a canal of stretchy muscle, 7.5–12 cm (3–5 in.) long, that connects the womb to the outside of the body. This soft, elasticated tube brings babies into the world and allows blood to exit your uterus during your period. It is also a key pleasure zone during sex, whether entered with fingers, toys or a penis. When aroused, the vagina may become "wet", lubricating itself more than usual in response to sexual excitement, which eases the friction of intercourse or foreplay, though not all vaginas respond to stimulation in this way.

The walls of the vagina are made up of many layers of tissue, similar to the inside lining of your mouth. Underneath these layers is collagen and the elastic fibres that give it the remarkable ability to both stretch to the size of a baby's head, and to tightly hold a tampon in place.

THE HYMEN IS A MARK OF VIRGINITY

The hymen is a very thin section of mucosal tissue found inside the opening of the vagina. Contrary to popular belief, it does not completely cover the vagina at all; instead, it's shaped like a bagel, with a slight opening that allows people to have periods, and the free flow of vaginal fluids before penetrative sex happens for the first time.

Perhaps the most persistent myth about the hymen is that it "breaks" the first time someone has sex, leading to the popular phrase "popping your cherry". In fact, though first sexual experiences can be uncomfortable, this is because of the hymen stretching and not because it has been "broken". Some people are born without a hymen at all, and for many, the hymen stretches long before they have sex for the first time, through sport or the natural growth of their body.

CREATING THE VAGINA

It is possible to have a vagina even if you were not born with one. For transgender people, whose sense of gender identity does not match the sex that they were assigned at birth, gender affirmation surgery can pave the way to a more complete sense of self.

Not all transgender women opt to undergo gender affirmation surgery for personal or financial reasons, and it is certainly not required in order for a transgender person's experience of womanhood to be valid or feel complete, but for many it can be a life-changing experience.

While the constructed vagina of a transgender woman will not connect to a female reproductive system, post-operative trans vaginas can still orgasm, experience penetrative sex and look largely indistinguishable from vaginas developed since birth.

It's important to know that asking a transgender person questions about their genitals is extremely rude. Whether they've undergone surgery or not is nobody's business but their own.

THE CERVIX

The cervix connects the vagina to the womb. The organ is divided into two: the ectocervix, which is the outer surface of the cervix, and the endocervix, which – you guessed it – is the inside of the cervix. The cervix is particularly important for people who menstruate as it opens each month to allow blood to flow out of the vagina during your period while the womb is shedding its lining.

During the ovulation stage of the menstrual cycle, the mucus produced by the cervix – which protects the womb, ovaries and fallopian tubes from infection – becomes thinner. This means that sperm can now travel up the fallopian tubes and fertilize the egg.

While a person is pregnant, their cervix closes to protect the baby, opening again at the moment of birth, when it dilates, meaning it stretches and softens, allowing the baby to leave the womb and enter the vaginal canal. The cervix opens up to an incredible 10 cm (4 in.) at the moment of birth, roughly the size of a large bagel.

THE UTERUS

Also known as the womb, the uterus plays a crucial role in the reproductive system. Around the size of a pear, it sits between the bladder and the rectum and its job is to take care of fertilized eggs until the foetus is ready to be birthed.

The uterus is made from three distinct layers: the outer protective layer; the myometrium, which forms the muscular middle layer; and the endometrium, which lines the womb. Either side of the top wall of the uterus, the fallopian tubes lead to the ovaries, allowing eggs to travel down into the womb. The lower part of the uterus connects to the cervix and so the vagina.

During ovulation, the endometrium walls of the uterus become thick and soft, ready to provide a pillowy home for a fertilized egg. If no such egg materializes, levels of progesterone and oestrogen drop, causing the uterus to contract and begin shedding its walls, resulting in a period.

THE FALLOPIAN TUBES

Fallopian tubes are the highways of the reproductive system: they allow eggs to pass from the ovaries to the womb. There are two fallopian tubes, one on each side of the womb, and they connect directly to the ovaries.

Each fallopian tube is around 10 cm (4 in.) long and slender, at around 7.5 mm (0.3 in.) in diameter. The egg is carried through the fallopian tubes to the uterus by small, hair-like linings. If the egg is fertilized by sperm during its journey, then sperm and egg will merge and begin to develop as they travel to the womb, eventually growing into a baby.

Fallopian tubes were named after the first person to describe them in detail, the sixteenth-century Italian master of anatomy, Gabriele Falloppio. He believed that they resembled tubas, which was mistranslated in English to form the "tube" part of the name.

This part of the reproductive system is extremely delicate, and can easily be impacted by sexually transmitted infections, pelvic inflammatory disease or endometriosis.

VAGINAL DISCHARGE MEANS SOMETHING IS WRONG

Worried about the discharge left in your pants after a long day? Don't be. Discharge is a completely normal part of everyday life and protects your vagina from infection while keeping it clean and moist. What amounts to a "normal" level of discharge differs for everyone. Much like sweat, some people will produce barely any while others will create several teaspoons a day. There is no right or wrong amount, whatever is normal for you is perfectly natural.

Your discharge will change significantly during different times of your cycle. During ovulation (approximately 14 days before your period), it may become sticky and you'll probably feel noticeably wetter. Right before ovulation, it'll be white and thick. After ovulation has finished, your discharge may be dry, or disappear completely.

The only time to worry about your discharge is if you notice a change in the usual smells, consistency or colour of your secretions. Then it's time to visit your doctor.

THE OVARIES

The ovaries are the primary sexual organ for those born with a vagina, and they play three very important roles – secreting hormones, releasing eggs for fertilization and protecting those eggs. If you were born with a vagina, then you already have all the eggs you will ever possess – it's the job of the ovaries to ensure they come to no harm.

Mature ovaries are the size of a large grape and are positioned on either side of the uterus, following on from the fallopian tubes. Ovaries produce hormones called oestrogen and progesterone as well as relaxin and inhibin. Oestrogen helps the body to develop "secondary sex" characteristics associated with the female body, including breasts and rounded, larger hips. Progesterone thickens the lining of the womb in order to make it receptive to a fertilized egg. Relaxin loosens pelvic ligaments to allow them to stretch during labour, and inhibin stops the pituitary gland from releasing any hormones. Before menopause, the ovaries also produce 50 per cent of the body's testosterone, which they release directly into the bloodstream.

The ovaries release one egg each menstrual cycle – this process is ovulation. Ovary-owners are born with between 150,000 and 500,000 eggs, though this drops to 34,000 by the time they are sexually mature. Only about 400 mature eggs will actually go through the ovulation process, and by the age of around 52, nearly all of the eggs are gone.

Before puberty, the ovaries are nothing more than a mass of tissue, and during menopause and beyond, they rapidly reduce in size, shrivelling to almost nothing, disappearing as magically as they arrived as they are no longer required by the body.

Some ovary-owners who are not yet ready to have children but want to ensure the option remains open to them as they age opt to undergo a process called "cryopreservation" in order to "freeze" their eggs. The procedure removes part of the ovary and freezes it, storing it in liquid nitrogen until it is required for fertilization.

THE VAGINA DURING MENOPAUSE

Menopause, the natural part of ageing when vagina-owners cease having periods, has a variety of effects on the vagina.

As the ovaries produce less oestrogen, the tissue and lining of the vagina often become thinner, less flexible and less lubricated. Known as "vaginal atrophy", this reduction in lubrication can be very uncomfortable. Thankfully, there are many solutions available through conversation with your doctor, including topical oestrogen therapy, which relieves the physical symptoms but doesn't allow the oestrogen to enter the bloodstream.

If vagina-owners aren't having much sexual activity during their menopause years, the vagina can also become shorter and narrower, which can cause pain when sexual activity is next attempted. A great way to avoid this if you aren't currently sharing sex with a partner is to enjoy moments of self-pleasure, discovering toys that, with the aid of lubricant, can keep your vagina flexible with the added benefit of making you feel great.

The most important thing for vagina-owners going through the menopause is to talk to their doctors about the changes they're experiencing. So many people don't get the help they need out of embarrassment, enduring discomfort that could be aided through simple medications.

If it makes you feel more comfortable, you are always entitled to request a female doctor. It may be useful before your visit to keep a list of the symptoms that you are experiencing in order to ensure you cover all the bases during your appointment. You can also simply hand your list to your doctor rather than talking through it point by point.

Remember – you can always ask for a second opinion. No doctor should tell you that your menopause symptoms are something that need to be accepted at a certain time of life. Persevere until you find a medical practitioner who will take your discomfort seriously – it's what you deserve.

PERIODS

Let's be real, nobody enjoys periods. But if you equip yourself with knowledge of what exactly is going on during that "time of the month", you may just discover a new-found respect for your days of crimson. This chapter will explain what happens during your monthly bleeds as well as exploring experiences of menstruation across the world.

WHAT ARE PERIODS?

Periods, or menstruation, are the time in the menstrual cycle when a uterus-owner bleeds from the vagina. Periods occur roughly every 28 days and can last anywhere from three to eight days, though everybody will have their own schedule. The average age for a first period is 12, but they can start at any time from eight to 15. Most people find they are bleeding with a regular schedule by the time they reach 18.

Bleeding is usually heaviest in the first few days of menstruation, when the blood will be bright red in colour. As the flow lessens, this colour will change to a pink or brown shade. It's common for a girl's first period to be distinctly darker in colour than her subsequent menstruations.

> During a whole period, no more than five to 12 teaspoons of blood are lost, though some people do experience far heavier periods, for which there is plentiful help and support available through your doctor – it's not something you simply need to accept.

WHY DO PERIODS HAPPEN?

Periods occur because the body needs to remove the lining built up in the womb during ovulation. This lining is developed in order to provide a cosy environment for a fertilized egg, should one make its way to the womb. If no egg appears, the lining must be shed, and the process begins again. The decrease in oestrogen created by the ovaries following ovulation causes the uterus to cramp, and this begins the shedding process through which the lining is released, along with mucus and blood, through the vagina.

Though periods can be uncomfortable and sometimes even painful, it can be helpful to view your monthly bleed as something of a cleansing or new beginning. Periods are your body's way of clearing out mess that it no longer needs – a kind of womb decluttering. Try to tap into this sense of new beginnings and you may soon find that your period no longer feels like a burden, but a reminder to take stock and refresh your life, as well as your body.

PERIODS CAN ATTRACT SHARKS

A myth most likely born of a fear of tampons and one too many screenings of *Jaws*. A surprising number of people believe that swimming in the ocean while menstruating can alert bloodthirsty sharks to your location. There are absolutely zero recorded cases of women attacked by sharks on account of their periods.

First, menses doesn't consist of pure blood in a way that could seriously be expected to leave a passing shark drooling. Menstrual fluid is made up of mucus, vaginal secretions and endometrial particles as well as blood and clots, all of which would significantly mask the scent of the blood. Second, the blood lost during your period isn't "flowing" as it could be in a serious ocean-borne injury. Rather, it's just being expelled from your uterus, and not in high quantities at that. The average period removes just 80 ml (3 fl oz.) of blood from the body in total, so the amount likely to be lost during a quick dip in the sea is seriously low.

THE MENSTRUAL CYCLE EXPLAINED

The menstrual cycle is the natural rhythm of a uterus-owner's body that makes pregnancy possible. It is controlled through the rise and fall in levels of oestrogen. The length of the menstrual cycle is different for everyone. Though the average cycle will span around 28 days, anything from 21 to 40 days is considered normal. The menstrual cycle can largely be broken down into four key stages:

1. MENSTRUATION

Also known as the period, during this stage of the menstrual cycle – which typically lasts between three to eight days – the lining of the uterus is shed from the body through the vagina.

2. THE FOLLICULAR PHASE

Beginning on the first day of the period, and ending with ovulation, this is when the pituitary gland releases a follicle-stimulating hormone that prompts the ovary to produce between five and 20 follicles, each containing an immature egg. Typically, all but one follicle die, while that one develops into a mature egg. This process also triggers the lining of the uterus to begin thickening, so that it's ready to host a fertilized egg.

3. OVULATION

This is the stage of the menstrual cycle when the person is most fertile – when a mature egg is released from the ovary. The egg is passed down the fallopian tube toward the womb. Unless it encounters sperm during the next 24 hours and is fertilized, it will die. If it is fertilized, it will continue its progress toward the uterus.

4. THE LUTEAL PHASE

Though the egg has left the ovaries in search of pastures new, the follicle in which it matured survives on the surface of the ovary. Over the next fortnight, it is transformed into a "corpus luteum", which releases progesterone and oestrogen. This cocktail of hormones keeps the uterus lining thick in hopes that a fertilized egg may stick to it and begin to grow. If it does, it will release its own hormones to keep the corpus luteum working. The corpus luteum will maintain the thickened lining throughout pregnancy. If no pregnancy occurs, it withers and dies. The drop in progesterone that follows triggers menstruation, and the cycle starts again.

WHAT IS PMS?

Ninety per cent of people with periods experience **PMS** (premenstrual syndrome), a condition affecting their emotions, health and behaviour in the run-up to menstruation. Between five and 11 days before your bleed, you may encounter acne, mood swings, cravings, breast tenderness, bloating, stomach pain, headaches, anxiety, a change in sex drive or trouble sleeping.

Surprisingly little is known about **PMS**, considering how many people are affected, but it has been suggested that these symptoms come about due to the hormonal changes involved in the menstrual cycle. The best solution is to look after yourself as best you can in the run-up to your period. Maintain a regular sleep schedule, get plenty of exercise, take painkillers if needed and allow yourself a treat or two. If your body is crying out for chips or chocolate, sometimes it's best to listen.

IT'S THE PLACE WHERE
ALL THE MOST PAINFUL
THINGS HAVE HAPPENED.
BUT IT HAS GIVEN ME
INDESCRIBABLE PLEASURE.

Madonna

If symptoms of **PMS** are unbearable, it could be a sign of premenstrual dysphoric disorder (see page 70), for which help can be obtained through your doctor. Don't be afraid to ask for support if you need it, as there are plenty of treatment options available.

WHY DO WE GET CRAMPS?

Though common, period cramps can be extremely painful and a difficult part of menstruation to navigate. After all, your daily schedule doesn't stop when your period comes, and it's not unusual to have to go about your normal day even when in distinct pain. Doctors at University College London recently proved that cramps can be as extreme as the pain associated with heart attacks, providing some long sought-after ammo for responding to those who dismiss cramps as "women's problems".

Period pains occur when the muscle wall of the uterus contracts more vigorously than usual to aid in the shedding of the womb lining. This contraction suppresses the oxygen supply to the uterus, triggering the tissues to release pain chemicals. While pain chemicals are being released, the body continues producing the chemical prostaglandins, which increase contractions, enhancing the pain.

Most period pain can be treated through painkillers, applying heat through a hot water bottle, warm baths or exercise. In recent years, forward-thinking sanitary brands such as DAYE have introduced CBD tampons that are claimed to reduce the pain of period cramps for their users.

SANITARY PRODUCTS: WHAT'S WHAT?

SANITARY TOWELS

Sanitary towels are absorbent strips placed in underwear to soak up blood loss. Pads need to be changed every three to four hours to reduce the risk of a rash or infection and to remain at optimal absorption. The first mass-produced sanitary pad was created in 1896, marking an end to the use of rags.

TAMPONS

Tampons are plugs of soft material inserted into the vagina. They come with or without applicators for ease of insertion and are attached to a string that hangs out of the vagina for easy removal. They should be changed every four to eight hours. Forms of tampons have been used for thousands of years – ancient Egyptians fashioned their own from papyrus plants.

MENSTRUAL CUPS

Though they may seem like new kids on the block, menstrual cups have been around since the 1930s. These small, silicone cups are inserted into the vagina, where they collect blood. Once removed and rinsed, they can be reused and last years. They've been shown to hold as much blood as three regular tampons and can be kept in place for 12 hours.

YOUR PERIOD AND THE ENVIRONMENT

Though sanitary products are an undeniable necessity, the items we currently use are placing a huge strain on the environment. The average person who bleeds uses a staggering 11,000 disposable menstrual products over their lifetime, and with some sanitary towels containing 90 per cent plastic, it's impossible to deny the dangers this disposable system is posing to our planet.

Thankfully, there is another way, and the period industry is rapidly adapting to create more sustainable solutions as we become more conscious of the way our sanitary choices are affecting the world around us.

The most environmentally friendly way to deal with period blood is to go for a reusable menstrual cup. Now so common they're available in most pharmacies, two years of using a menstrual cup would save the equivalent of 528 disposable pads or tampons. Ten years of using these cups would save an entire truckload of waste from being dumped into the environment: Sir David Attenborough would be proud.

If you prefer to use tampons, avoiding disposable applicators will reduce the amount of plastic wasted. Tampons are available without applicators if you're comfortable using your fingers. If not, consider purchasing a reusable applicator that need simply be rinsed and reused. There are also plenty of organic tampon options on the market that are gentler on your vagina, reducing dryness and irritation.

Reusable pads can also be purchased, as can "period pants" – super-absorbent underwear that is leak-proof, remains dry to the touch and can simply be washed and reworn. Reusable pads can even be home-made; search online for a step-by-step guide. With so many options available, often proving kinder to the wallet as well as the planet, there's no excuse to shy away from having an eco-friendly period.

If you want to help your fellow vagina-owners as well as the planet, there are now many charities with the goal of alleviating period poverty. Close to 12 million women in the US and one in ten girls in the UK are unable to afford adequate sanitary products. Visit actionaid.org.uk to donate to people experiencing period poverty around the world.

PERIOD PROBLEMS

Periods are unpleasant at the best of times, but some people experience complications that make their monthly bleed even more stressful. Here are some of the most common:

PAINFUL BLEEDS

While cramps are a normal part of menstruation, for some people these pains can become severe enough to impact their daily life. If this sounds familiar, book an appointment with your doctor, who can suggest methods of pain reduction to make your period more manageable.

IRREGULAR BLEEDS

No idea when your next period will strike? If you experience dramatic variation in when your period occurs or in how much blood you lose, it's time to check it with your doctor. It's also crucial to seek medical advice if your periods stop completely.

PREMENSTRUAL DYSPHORIC DISORDER

If your PMS symptoms feel extreme, causing deep depressive feelings, irritability or wild mood swings, visit a doctor. You may be suffering with PDD, a severe version of PMS symptoms that affects up to 5 per cent of people who menstruate. Treatment can be offered in the form of antidepressants or birth control containing drospirenone or ethinyl estradiol.

YOU SHOULDN'T HAVE SEX DURING YOUR PERIOD

With cramps, stomach ache, increased hunger and irritability, the last thing you should have to do during your time of the month is deny yourself sex too! It's perfectly safe to engage in any of your regular sexual activities during your period, so if you and your partner feel comfortable with the possibility of slightly messier lovemaking, go for it. It might even aid your PMS, as orgasms have been shown to ease cramps by releasing tension in the muscles of the uterus.

Period sex has also been shown to make your periods shorter, provide natural lubrication and ease migraines, and many people report a higher sex drive during that time of the month. If you plan to experiment with a little scarlet sex, make sure you still use protection, as your period doesn't make you immune to sexually transmitted diseases or the possibility of getting pregnant.

**EVERY WOMAN'S BODY
IS DIFFERENT AND DEALS
WITH PAIN, CRAMPS,
BLEEDING DIFFERENTLY.
SO WORK OUT WHAT
IS BEST FOR YOU.**

Jessie J

SHADES OF GREY

Social media and tabloid inches have been awash in recent years with debate around the language we use to talk about periods. Conservative voices have vocally resisted the move of sanitary brands and period campaigners to replace the word "women" in their communications with "people who menstruate". But despite outrage from some, this was an important step to take.

To define everyone who menstruates as a "woman" is to ignore swathes of nuance in our experiences with both menstruation and gender. For many people with vaginas, menstruation is not part of their experience. For numerous cisgendered women (those who were born with female reproductive organs and identify as women), menstruation is not a part of their lives. Whether through health issues, menopause or medications, periods simply do not factor into their monthly cycles, and that's okay! It doesn't make them any less womanly.

Furthermore, these kinds of assertions allow no room for the many shades of grey in the spectrum of gender identity. Transgender women do not experience periods, but their experience of womanhood is just as valid and worthy as those who do. Transgender men may still experience monthly bleeding, but this does not stop them from being men, or render their experience of manhood less valid.

Rather than clamour to all be identified under a single umbrella, let's celebrate the wonderful diversity in the experiences of "womanhood" and "manhood" and see our differences as part of a unique and beautiful tapestry, rather than deviations from a dull one-size-fits-all norm.

The idea that we should say always "woman" instead of "people who menstruate" doesn't stack up for a very clear reason: not every woman bleeds, and not everybody who bleeds is a woman. Simple.

PERIODS AROUND THE WORLD

Monthly bleeds look very different in different parts of the world...

SOMALIA

Ninety-nine per cent of Somali people identify as Muslim and observe very strict rules around their time of the month. While bleeding, you cannot pray, fast or visit the mosque. It isn't permitted to follow the usual rules of the faith because during the week of your bleed, you are considered *dahir*, unclean. Once the period ceases, you must shower and wash your hair. Once the body is "purified", normal life may resume.

CANADA

For members of the Cree First Nation group, menstruation is known by another name: Moontime. The monthly cycle is seen as a gift from nature, during which time you are cleansed mentally, physically and spiritually. During their periods, Cree people are not expected to undertake any chores and are supported by family and friends so that they can instead use the time as a moment of reflection and self-renewal.

NEPAL

Nepalese culture can be unforgiving during the week of menstruation. Although it was outlawed in 2005, many communities persist in a practice known as Chaupadi, where the "unclean" menstruater is sent to live outside of the home, in a hut, cowshed or other outbuilding, regardless of the weather, often in extremely dangerous circumstances. It is thought that the monthly bleed offends Hindu gods and will bring a curse upon the house if they remain indoors.

JAPAN
Bleeding in Japan can have some unexpected consequences when it comes to your career. Tradition dictates that women cannot be sushi chefs, because periods throw off their sense of taste.

AFGHANISTAN
Rates of period poverty are particularly bad in Afghanistan, where 62 per cent of schoolgirls resort to using strips of clothing as they are unable to afford sanitary products. Menstruation is extremely taboo, and not to be discussed, which causes a range of issues. One particularly damaging belief sees people avoid washing their vaginas while menstruating, fearing that it can lead to infertility. Addressing the situation in Afghanistan is a key focus for charities such as World Vision International.

WHAT IS THE MENOPAUSE?

Monthly bleeding is not a lifelong state of affairs. Just as your period arrives in your teenage years, so it disappears between the ages of 45 and 55, though not without a fight.

Periods stop when levels of oestrogen in the body decline. As bleeds become less frequent, other symptoms of the menopause's arrival emerge, often causing considerable discomfort for the person going through "the change". Here are the most common:

HOT FLUSHES

Often accompanied by a quickened pulse, hot flushes are sudden feelings of heat that take over the body. Most vagina-owners find they subside by themselves, but in severe cases, hormone replacement therapy (HRT) can be used to put an end to flushes.

VAGINAL DRYNESS (AKA VAGINAL ATROPHY)

Over half of post-menopausal people experience vaginal dryness, caused by dropping oestrogen levels in the body. This can cause itching, burning and discomfort during sex. Treatments include personal lubricants and oestrogen tablets/creams applied to the vagina.

ANXIETY OR MOOD SWINGS

Higher stress levels, depression, anxiety and panic attacks are all common during menopausal years, enhanced by physical side effects such as sleeplessness and hormone fluctuation. Regular exercise can ease these symptoms, but if mental health concerns begin to impact your daily life, speak to your doctor to access treatment.

LIFE AFTER MENOPAUSE?

Although the symptoms of menopause can sometimes be hard to cope with, once their monthly bleeds are behind them, many people feel better than ever post-menopause and cite a renewed sense of well-being. According to a survey by *Health Plus* magazine, eight in ten post-menopausal people said they felt an "overwhelming sense of freedom" and ten years younger than before.

There are many reasons to celebrate putting your bleeding days behind you: no more **PMS**, monthly bloating, cravings or unexpected underwear-ruining. Plus, you'll be saving money on sanitary products, an expense that sets vagina-owners back more than £18,000 in the course of their lifetimes.

Perhaps most excitingly, post-menopause you have increased control over your body. With the threat of unwanted pregnancy and the monthly cycle of periods in your past, your body belongs entirely to you, and is yours to use as you wish. This is a great chance to take stock of your life and health and put steps in place to care for yourself better than ever before.

SEX

Time for the fun bit. Yes, your vagina performs a lot of vital functions within the body, but it's also your playground, capable of delivering knee-shaking orgasms and scintillating sensations. Whether you gratify your desires alone, with a toy or with a partner, here's everything you need to know about taking your vagina to pleasure town.

LOVE YOURSELF FIRST

We don't *think* drag superstar RuPaul was talking about masturbation when they said, "If you can't love yourself, how in the hell you gonna love somebody else?", but if they were, they weren't wrong. Despite centuries of stigma, taboo and shame, let us declare it once and for all – there is absolutely no downside, danger or damage associated with masturbation. It's natural, it's healthy, and it feels great! If masturbation feels good for you, then masturbate.

Masturbation offers a host of health benefits, from relieving period pains to reducing stress and improving sleep quality. Some experts have even claimed that it aids in faster recovery from sickness, as it increases the body's production of white blood cells. And a *ménage à moi* won't just benefit your health. Regular masturbation increases your chances of orgasm with a partner and improves sexual confidence.

There's no right or wrong position to enjoy your me-time. Some people lie on their back, some kneel, some lie on their front. If it feels good, you're doing it right. Enjoy...

PLEASURE ZONES

Pleasure is often simplified to two zones: the vagina for penetration and the clitoris for stimulation. The reality is that the vagina is even more committed to your pleasure, with six different zones all geared up to provide killer orgasms, if you just know how to arouse them.

VAGINAL ENTRY

The first few centimetres of the vaginal canal are extremely sensitive. Pay extra attention to this area and fireworks will soon fly.

THE G-SPOT

Part of the clitoral network, stimulation of the G-spot is actually stimulation of the clitoris from inside the vagina. Properly aroused – researchers have suggested that replicating a "come hither" action with fingers has the best results – this humble spot can lead to big orgasms or even the elusive female ejaculation.

LOTS OF SEX MAKES VAGINAS "LOOSE"

A myth used to slut-shame sexually promiscuous women for centuries, the idea that engaging in lots of sexual activity results in a loose or saggy vagina is completely false.

Society perpetuates many falsities when it comes to the tightness – or lack thereof – of the vagina. First, that virgins have particularly tight vaginas, loosened by their first sexual experience. Second, that frequent sex loosens it further. Third, that childbirth loosens the vagina to an extent that it can never recover. None of these rumours are true.

Vaginas are extremely elastic. They're also a "potential space", which means that they aren't open at all most of the time. The resting vagina measures between 5 and 10 cm (2–4 in.) but can stretch to almost magic proportions, Transformer-style, to a circumference of 10 cm (4 in.) during childbirth. Despite this incredible change, it can snap back to its original shape very quickly: most birthing bodies find that their vagina has returned to its former size within six months of childbirth.

DEEP SPOT UPPER

A favourite among truly intrepid vagina explorers, the "deep spot upper" can be discovered on the upper wall around a centimetre below the point where the vagina meets the cervix. Stimulated during deep penetration, the sensations can be extremely intense.

DEEP SPOT LOWER

This pleasure zone resides at the same depth as the deep spot upper, but involves stimulation of the lower wall of the vagina instead. This sweet spot can be stimulated through both vaginal and anal play.

CERVIX

Perhaps the most surprising spot on the list, for some people stimulation of the cervix is the height of sexual pleasure. You can find this spot by entering the vagina as far as possible. At the very top is the cervix. Beware, though – this spot is certainly not everybody's cup of sexual tea, so proceed with caution.

THE CLITORIS

Also known as the "devil's doorbell", "love button" and "sweet spot", for most vagina-owners the clitoris is the key to sexual success. Though myths of its elusive nature persist, it's actually very easy to locate, at the top of the vulva, covered with its clitoral hood. While some people enjoy direct stimulation, for others the feelings are so intense they cause discomfort, and concentrating on the surrounding area is the secret to reaching orgasm. There's only one way to discover your own preference, and practice makes perfect!

THE BIOLOGY OF THE ORGASM

Described variously as a sensation of electricity, freefalling, relief or bliss, a vagina-owner's orgasm serves no reproductive purpose, unlike the penile orgasm, but seems to exist for pleasure's sake alone. So, what's actually happening when you reach the big O?

- When you become aroused by stimuli, whether physical, visual or audible, blood flow to the vagina increases, which causes it to become more sensitive. As you become more turned on, your heart rate, blood pressure and rate of breathing also increase. At this time, the clitoris becomes erect and engorged by the blood flow, and the vagina becomes more lubricated.

- When you reach the height of sensitivity, the muscles of the vagina and uterus begin to produce intensely powerful rhythmic contractions that release the muscle tension that built up during arousal, causing that overwhelming feeling of "letting go".

- As your heart rate drops and breathing returns to normal, it's common to feel extremely sleepy following a knee-shaking orgasm. Many vagina-owners can proceed to have multiple orgasms if stimulation continues, while for others the heightened sensitivity means that continued stimulation becomes uncomfortable.

THE ORGASM GAP

The "orgasm gap" is a term used to describe the disparity that exists between the orgasms of heterosexual men and women. According to a recent Durex study, three in four women don't always orgasm during sex and 20 per cent of women don't experience orgasm at all. One in five women in the same study said that their partner didn't do the right things to bring them to orgasm.

A 2016 study by the Archives of Sexual Behaviour, meanwhile, found that 95 per cent of men said that they always orgasmed during sex, compared to just 65 per cent of women. Heterosexual women were found to be the least likely to experience orgasm during a sexual experience.

Professor Laura Mintz of the University of Florida claims that this is down to our "cultural ignorance of the clitoris". So how do we get past this, and ensure that we get the orgasms we deserve?

Well, if you have the script for a movie or TV show that showcases the orgasm gap in all its glory, get it out there! More realistic depictions of orgasms – or lack thereof – are sorely needed if we are to beat the pervading view that all we need for a world-ending O is a few thrusts of James Bond's golden gun.

When it comes to your personal orgasm-gap battlefield, the solution is simple. Whatever your sexuality, the key to a heart-shattering orgasm is the same: communication.

I WISH EVERYBODY COULD
TALK ABOUT THE GENITAL
TRACT IN THE SAME WAY
WE TALK ABOUT THE
ELBOW OR THE FOOT.
IT'S JUST A BODY PART.

Jen Gunter

Does the way your partner is touching you feel good? Tell them! Not working for you? Tell them – or even better, show them – what would make you feel good instead.

There's nothing sexier than making someone else feel good in the bedroom, so speak up. Not only will communicating what you want make you far more likely to reach orgasm, but it will also make the experience more enjoyable for your partner, as they get to see you in the throes of true pleasure, and even help you get there!

CONTRACEPTION: WHAT'S WHAT

Contraception serves two purposes – to protect you from sexually transmitted diseases and prevent unwanted pregnancies. Here are some of the most popular forms of contraceptive.

SHORT-TERM CONTRACEPTION

CONDOMS

Condoms place a physical barrier – usually latex or polyurethane – between ejaculate and the cervix. They also protect both partners against STDs.

- **How to use:** Remove the condom from the packet, taking care not to rip the material. Squeeze the teat to remove any air, and place over the head of the penis, rolling the condom down to cover it. Post-ejaculation, it's important that the wearer holds the base of the condom firmly to ensure it doesn't come off inside the vagina.

- **Pros:** 98 per cent effective protection against both pregnancy and STDs.

- **Cons:** Can split or tear if not used correctly.

DENTAL DAM

These thin latex sheets can be placed over the vagina during oral sex to protect both the wearer and giver from sexual transmitted infections.

- **Pros:** Makes oral sex enjoyable without the risk of STDs.

- **Cons:** Can reduce sensitivity.

DIAPHRAGM

Place this silicone "cap" into your vagina before sex, pushed up against the cervix, and it will act as a barrier between sperm and your uterus.

- **Pros:** 92–96 per cent effective hormone-free protection against pregnancy.

- **Cons:** The cap must be kept in place for at least six hours after sex to ensure effectiveness. It doesn't protect against STDs.

THE PATCH

Similar in appearance to a nicotine patch, these adhesive squares slowly release oestrogen and progesterone into the bloodstream. Patches can be worn anywhere on the body and should be changed once a week.

- **Pros:** 99 per cent effective against pregnancy, only need to be changed once a week and can help regulate periods.

- **Cons:** Patches don't protect against STDs.

LONG-TERM CONTRACEPTION

THE COIL

Also known as IUDs, these T-shaped copper devices are placed into the uterus by a doctor or nurse. The slow release of copper alters the mucus in the cervix, making it more difficult for sperm to survive.

- **Pros:** 99 per cent effective against pregnancy and can last for up to ten years.

- **Cons:** Some women find insertion uncomfortable, and they don't protect against STDs.

THE PILL

These tiny tablets contain artificial versions of oestrogen and progesterone. This hormone cocktail stops ovaries from releasing eggs, thickens the mucus in the neck of the womb so it's harder to penetrate, and thins the lining of the womb, making it less hospitable for any egg warriors that overcome these other obstacles. A pill is taken every day for 21 days, followed by a seven-day break in which the user experiences their bleed.

- **Pros:** The pill is 99 per cent effective against unwanted pregnancy. Some women report additional benefits, including reduced acne and regular periods.

- **Cons:** A wide variety of side effects are possible, including headaches, weight gain or a change in libido. The pill doesn't protect against STDs.

THE "MINI PILL"

The progesterone-only pill doesn't contain oestrogen and works by thickening the mucus in the cervix, making it harder for sperm to travel. This pill needs to be taken every day for its 99 per cent effectiveness.

- **Pros:** Protects against pregnancy, is oestrogen-free and can reduce heavy periods.

- **Cons:** Doesn't protect against STDs and can cause side effects such as mood changes, nausea or acne in some women.

THE IMPLANT

This humble device sounds far scarier than it actually is. A small plastic rod is fitted under the skin of your upper arm with the help of local anaesthetic. For three years, it will release progesterone to protect you from pregnancy, with a 99 per cent effectiveness rate.

- **Pros:** Can be removed at any time and may stop periods completely.

- **Cons:** Side effects can include nausea, headaches and acne. Implants don't protect against STDs.

THE INJECTION

The progesterone released through the hormone injection is effective for between eight and 13 weeks, depending on brand, and is a popular choice for people who find they forget to take the pill.

- **Pros:** Offers 99 per cent effective protection against pregnancy.

- **Cons:** The injection doesn't protect against STDs, and it can take up to a year for fertility to return to normal after stopping injections.

PULL-OUT METHOD

Just kidding. Withdrawing the penis before ejaculation is *not an effective contraceptive method*. Please don't rely on this.

- **Pros:** No pros.
- **Cons:** Offers zero protection against STDs or unwanted pregnancy.

"SQUIRTING" DURING SEX IS JUST PEE

Not every vagina-owner experiences "squirting" during sex – a moment when fluid is rapidly expelled at the point of orgasm – but for those who do it can be surprising, and sometimes embarrassing. Perhaps you hadn't heard of squirting before experiencing it or, even worse, perhaps you feared you'd simply had an accident.

Squirting is nothing more than an exciting response to some seriously good stimulation, and nothing to be ashamed of. And that fluid is certainly not urine, though the pre-climax feeling has been described as similar to the sensation of needing to pee. When you use the toilet, urine leaves the bladder through the urethra. When you squirt, the glands *around* the urethra gush secretions out in time with an orgasm. This fluid is clear, not yellow, and doesn't smell like pee either.

Scientific research by sexologist Beverly Whipple in the 1980s found that pee particles were present in extremely low amounts in squirt fluid; and in fact the fluid contained a substance known as PSA (prostate-specific antigen), which is also produced in the male prostate gland.

TALKING ABOUT SEX

The short cut to a fulfilling sex life? It's about more than one pair of lips. Get communicating about your sexual needs and desires and you'll soon find that you're experiencing sex with more confidence and understanding of what it is you really want.

Talking to your partner openly will ensure that they know just what to do to please you. And you may even find some hidden desires that make themselves known once you start talking.

It's time to end the culture of "faking orgasms". If your partner isn't getting you there, then tell them what *will* get you off, or show them how you get there yourself. Faking your orgasm doesn't help anyone. It won't help your partner to please you in the future, it won't get you the orgasm you deserve, and it'll only increase the pressure you feel to "orgasm" every time. There are no Oscars for faking it.

For most vagina-owners, orgasm is not going to be possible with *every* sexual encounter, but open communication is the best way to feel good, even if that doesn't involve the big O.

HOW TO TALK ABOUT SEX

TALK TO YOURSELF FIRST

Listen to how your body is feeling during different sexual experiences. Ask yourself, *when is sex good for me? When do I feel unsatisfied? What would I like to explore? What am I certain I don't like?* It might be helpful to practise your conversation beforehand with a friend, or even by yourself.

START THE CONVERSATION

If you're uncomfortable asserting your desires, try asking questions instead. "Would you be interested in trying __?", "I'd like to establish a safe word. Would __ work?" When you're ready, use phrases such as: "I really like it when you __" or "I don't think __ works for me."

PRACTICE MAKES PERFECT

Great sex can't come from one conversation alone – it should be a constant dialogue between you and your partner(s). Address things that make you uncomfortable or new fantasies you discover, and remember, there is absolutely nothing wrong with communicating your needs.

The final secret? Listening! Ask your partner about what they enjoy too. Mind-blowing sex takes two!

PLAY TIME: SEX TOYS

Toys can serve a variety of purposes during a healthy, happy sex life. Struggle to reach orgasm? They're about to become your best friend. Want to add some variety to your sex life? They're the perfect solution.

Sex toys are becoming more popular, with the global market worth a staggering $48.2 billion. The BBC recently reported that 70 per cent of Europeans and 60–65 per cent of women in the US own sex toys, though some states, including Alabama and Texas, still have draconian laws preventing their sale. Not only does this encourage a culture of shame, but it also discriminates against people for whom physical intimacy isn't possible without aids.

If you're lucky enough to live somewhere that sex toys are legal, make the most of it! And if the very thought of a sex store brings to mind intimidating images of gimp suits and enormous dildos, fear not. Not only is it easy and discreet to shop online, but sex toys also come in all shapes and sizes, from tiny vibrators to crystal wands, so there's sure to be something out there to tickle your fanny... sorry... fancy.

FOUR ORGASMIC SEX POSITIONS

Let's face it. Some sexual positions just aren't going to get you there when it comes to reaching your *petite mort*. Here are some go-to limb tangles for maximum pleasure.

SPOONS
Best for: Intimate stimulation
Position yourself either lying down or seated with your partner behind you acting as the big spoon. With this increased access, they can explore you with their hands, offering intimate kisses or strokes to your back, neck and face in the process. If they have a penis or toys, they can penetrate in this position to up the intensity. You can also add a vibrator in front to offer some additional stimulation.

ON TOP
Best for: Complete control
Straddle your partner while they lie on their back so that they can penetrate you using toys, hands or their penis

from below. As you're on top, you can control the depth, angle and speed of movement, and add in your own hands or toys to increase your chance of reaching orgasm. To stimulate your G-spot, lean back slightly as you move.

COITAL ALIGNMENT TECHNIQUE
Best for: Grinding action

Sure, it's not the sexiest name, but this position can work wonders. Lie on your back in traditional missionary position, with your partner on top. They should shift themselves up so that their penis, toy or hands, are slightly higher up than usual. Then, instead of thrusting in and out, they should use a grinding motion against your pelvis. If the angle isn't working, try popping a pillow or two under your hips.

ORAL SEX
Best for: Orgasms on orgasms

Oral sex might just have the highest hit rate when it comes to achieving orgasms, though everyone has their own style. You might prefer to be on your knees, to be stimulated from behind, or to lie on your back. However you're positioned, make sure you're comfortable and remember it's not a race. Focus on enjoying the journey rather than the end goal and you'll soon find yourself in bliss. And don't forget, communication is sexy! Let your partner know as soon as they've found your sweet spot.

PORNOGRAPHIC PUSSY

We all have nights where that perfectly steamy masturbation inspiration just won't strike, and for some people, the solution is pornography. If that's you, no shame! There's nothing wrong with enjoying some fun between consenting adults. In fact, 35 per cent of all content downloaded from the internet is pornographic in nature, and it's estimated that some 28,000 users are watching pornography every second.

If you're consuming pornographic content, it's really important to remember that the bodies and scenarios you're watching do not reflect real life. Lighting, scripting, strategic editing – and even plastic surgery – are relied upon by the porn industry to create the "perfect" sexual fantasies that play out on your screen. In real life, things tend to be a lot messier – and that's half the fun! Certainly, the performances given by stars of the business in no way represent a "standard" that you should endeavour to replicate. There is no one way to be sexy and no one way to engage in sex.

MIRROR MIRROR

So many vagina-owners are held back in the bedroom by a lack of self-esteem. And based on the 44 per cent of women who couldn't identify the vagina on a medical diagram, many of us are self-conscious about an area we've never properly seen!

Grab yourself a mirror, open those pins and take a good look at your vagina. Gently spread your labia and take in its delicate shape and deep colours. This is you, and you are absolutely perfect.

Not only is looking at your vagina empowering, but it's also key for keeping on top of your health. It's really important to know what is normal for you, and to have a good knowledge of how your vagina looks, so you'll be quick to notice when something has gone awry.

PEOPLE HAVE TO START RESPECTING THE VAGINA.

Janelle Monáe

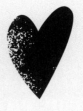

VAGINAS IN CULTURE

Ah, culture and the vagina. Films where a few thrusts from the hero has women collapsing in orgasmic bliss. Nude statues with vaginas as smooth as an egg. Songs that describe good sex as painful sex. But it's not all bad. A new generation of artists are going out of their way to repaint the vagina in film, books and music using all the colours of the rainbow – and we're here for it.

YOU NEED SPECIAL PRODUCTS
TO CLEAN THE VAGINA

Despite the wealth of products on offer promising to clean and restore balance to your downstairs, you do not need to use anything specific when washing your nether regions. In fact, using soaps and shower gels anywhere inside your labia majora can be extremely bad for your vaginal health, leading to a pH imbalance and all manner of infections.

One of the many wonders of the vagina is that it's self-cleaning. Your regular secretions see to the cleaning and maintenance of your vagina all by themselves, without the aid of perfumed soaps or wipes.

When showering, simply use an unscented soap to gently wash around the outside of the vulva and your perineal area, between the vagina and anus. Douching – the process of flushing water up into the vagina to clear out secretions – can disrupt your natural bacteria, leading to yet more infections and is completely unnecessary for keeping your vagina clean.

THE ART OF THE VAGINA

The very first artistic depiction of a vagina was inscribed into a rockface in France in around 35,000 BC. Stone Age art is rife with fertility symbols, often expressed in figurines of women with highly exaggerated curves and vaginas. By the time of the ancient Romans, this artistic celebration of the vagina had changed. Nude statues in ancient Rome don't depict female genitals, presenting suspiciously smooth stone in place of the lips of the labia. Of course, the same rule of modesty was not applied when chiselling their male counterparts. The vagina, and representations of female sexuality, were already being considered "obscene" and erased from the cultural discourse. As Jane Caputi writes in her book, *Goddesses and Monsters* "while the phallus is deified, its female symbolic equivalent [...] is everywhere stigmatized".

Thankfully this has not remained the case. In 1866, Gustave Courbet painted his hugely controversial work, *The Origin of the World* – a close-up of a woman's vagina as she reclines. The painting isn't pornographic, but frank, daring and commanding. Today, the painting is the second highest selling postcard at the Musée d'Orsay, where it now resides.

The following three artworks each offered a groundbreaking depiction of a vagina. Have a Google or undertake your own pussy pilgrimage to explore these remarkable creations.

Hon-en Katedral / Niki de Saint Phalle, Per Olof Ultvedt and Jean Tinguely / 1966

This huge, reclining figure was a painted in a rainbow of patterns, her legs spread, her vagina a doorway to several interior rooms, including a cinema and a milk bar in the right breast. The 28-m-long (92-ft) sculpture served to insist, very physically, on the importance of centring the work of women in our museums and galleries.

The Dinner Party / Judy Chicago / 1979

Housed in Brooklyn Museum, this notorious installation by feminist artist Judy Chicago takes the form of a large triangular table, with place settings reserved for 39 famous women. Each setting represents a uniquely designed vagina, laid out for such guests as Virginia Woolf, Susan B. Anthony and Boadicea.

***Diva* / Juliana Notari / 2021**

There's nothing subtle about this vagina: bright red, constructed from reinforced concrete and measuring 33 m (108 ft), Juliana Notari's *Diva* adorns the hillside of a rural park in Brazil.

CLITERARY HISTORY

Vaginas haven't had the easiest ride in literature, particularly when it comes to early Christian writings. "Woman is the gate to hell and her gaping genitals the yawning mouth of hell," said Tertullian, an author writing in the second century AD who also dubbed the vagina the "devil's doorway". He probably didn't intend that to sound quite as cool as it does.

Meanwhile, the ancient Roman senator Boethius wrote that "Woman is a temple built on a sewer", and Catholic saint Odo of Cluny declared that "To embrace a woman is to embrace a sack of manure." Delightful.

No wonder then, that American playwright Eve Ensler opened her infamous off-Broadway show *The Vagina Monologues* in 1996 with the words: "My vagina's angry.

It's pissed off. My vagina's furious and it needs to talk. It needs to talk about all this shit. It needs to talk to you."

The script was inspired by interviews with vagina-owners from all walks of life and, while it touches on the violence performed against vaginas across the world, it also celebrates the joy a healthy relationship with your down-there can create.

Thankfully the attitudes of the early centuries AD didn't prevail. As the years wore on, outlooks began to change, and today you can discover a multitude of writings about the vagina that are both positive and educational. The Further Reading list on page 142 is a great place to start.

From the sixties and seventies, women's magazines began to be more open about sexuality. One title in particular grew to become a self-styled sex bible – *Cosmopolitan*. Though founded in 1886, *Cosmo* as we know it came to life in 1965 under the helm of Helen Gurley Brown, who reinvented the mag as a racy handbook for the busy career woman. *Cosmo*'s frank discussions of sex made it immensely popular – though not with some feminists, who symbolically dumped copies of the magazine into a "freedom trash can" during protests at the 1968 Miss America pageant.

Today, there is more frank discussion of the vagina than ever before, and even, for the first time, a museum in its honour. London's Vagina Museum opened its doors in 2019 with a mission to educate and advocate for an inclusive and intersectional perspective on the vagina.

SILVER SCREEN SNATCH

Perhaps surprisingly, the genre to speak most explicitly about the vagina through cinematic history has been horror. While romantic films may lean on the tasteful pan away at their stars' most intimate moments, horror movies have frequently placed the vagina centre stage. In these films, it becomes a symbol of frightening power.

In the 1976 adaptation of Stephen King's *Carrie*, a teen develops terrifying powers with the dawn of her period. *Poltergeist* (1982) has its victims sucked into another dimension through a fleshy vagina-esque hole in the wall. Then 1990 brought us *Predator 2*, where the alien antagonist is dubbed "pussy face" by one of their unfortunate victims, and in 2007's *Teeth* the heroine's vagina is lined with its own set of pearly whites, ready to savage those who dare cross her.

Throughout the decades, the vagina on screen has held the power to scare and enthral in equal measure. But audiences' thirst for stories that show the vagina's power with the sense of reverence that it deserves remains unsated.

Vaginas that spark fear? Sure, that's easy to come by. But films where women's desire is the main theme? That's a little trickier. It says something that perhaps the most famous female orgasm scene of all time doesn't involve an orgasm at all, thanks to Meg Ryan's exceptional "faking it" skills in *When Harry Met Sally* (1989).

In recent years a spate of films has thankfully begun to challenge this. French romance *A Portrait of a Lady on Fire* (2019) and English historical drama *The Favourite* (2018) both tenderly explore the intimacy of lesbian sex in a tasteful yet defiantly frank nature.

Representations of cunnilingus on screen are on the rise. In *Blue Valentine* (2010), Ryan Gosling's character doesn't hesitate to give some oral pleasure to his partner, though it didn't delight the ratings board, earning the film an 18/NC-17 rating. Meanwhile, in Netflix's wildly successful period drama series *Bridgerton* (2020), cunnilingus is a regular feature in the frolics of the Duke of Hastings and Daphne's adventurous sex life, much to its audience's delight.

VAGINAS ON THE SMALL SCREEN

Perhaps no television show has done quite so much to put vaginas at the forefront of its agenda than *Sex and the City*. Running for six seasons from 1998 until 2004, the show unashamedly spoke about the vaginas and desires of its four stars, in particular Samantha Jones, the sexual savant who declared, "My vagina waits for no man."

Many of the storylines from this iconic show are far from feminist when viewed in a modern context, but without doubt, *SATC* revolutionized the way that vagina-owners were depicted on our screens. Over the course of six seasons, viewers tuned into 96 sex scenes replete with STDs, disappointing lovers, health scares and, of course, knee-knocking orgasms.

The show was designed to appeal to the generation of women who "had it all", juggling holding down successful careers, enjoying exciting sex, dressing like fashionistas and starting families. Though very much of its time, *Sex and the City*'s influence can still be felt today, with shows such as *Girls* and *Broad City* undoubtedly owing something of their success to the blueprint laid down by Carrie and the girls.

TV representation is on the up. One of those shows indebted to *Sex and the City*, *Broad City* (2009), found its niche in the surprisingly wholesome comedic value of its stars' relationships with their vaginas.

Meanwhile, the Netflix original cartoon *Big Mouth* (2017), which centres around a group of teenagers as they undergo the wild years of puberty, has entire episodes dedicated to periods, the vagina and masturbation. Indeed, one of the lead characters, Jesi, has a vagina that is a character in its own right, voiced by Kristen Wiig. Talking to her owner for the first time, Jesi's vagina gives her a grand tour, asking "Have you ever been electrocuted, but in a good way?" as she introduces the clit.

Another Netflix original, *Sex Education* (2019) – which also follows a group of teenagers coping with the trials and joys of their changing bodies – covers topics including sexually transmitted diseases, masturbation, sex and leaked nudes.

MAKING SWEET MUSIC

Music videos have been a frontier for vagina representation in recent years. Take Ariana Grande's "God is a Woman" (2018) for example, where the singer sits with the world quite literally between her thighs, swims in a pool shaped like a vulva and is even at one point backed by a chorus of singing beavers.

Meanwhile Janelle Monae's "PYNK" (2018) sees the singer and her backing dancers bedecked in vulva-like trousers and fondling suggestive slices of fruit, surrounded by boxes of oysters, furry kitties and underwear emblazoned with phrases like "sex cells" and "pussy power".

In the video for "WAP" by Cardi B and Megan Thee Stallion (2020), water gushes down the corridors of an ornate manor, where wild cats roam the halls and rooms are lined with bouquets of flowers.

And in Miley Cyrus' "Mother's Daughter" (2020), the singer shows close-ups of pants holding pads and lips blowing bubble-gum bubbles while sporting a red leather catsuit with toothed vagina decal. The message is clear: this pussy grabs back.

A PUSSY PLAYLIST

There can be great empowerment to be found in lyrics about the vagina. Whether you're dancing to Charli XCX, bopping to Cyndi Lauper or rapping along with Doja Cat, pour a drink and turn the volume up for your very own pussy party.

"Soft as Snow" by My Bloody Valentine
"Peaches and Cream" by 112
"She Bop" by Cyndi Lauper
"Work It" by Missy Elliot
"Body of My Own" by Charli XCX
"I Love Me" by Hailee Steinfeld
"Kicks" by FKA Twigs
"Doves in the Wind" by SZA ft Kendrick Lamar

"Go to Town" by Doja Cat
"I Can't" by Foxy Brown

WHAT IS FEMINISM?

Feminism is a movement that advocates for the social, political and economic equality of the sexes. True feminism is intersectional, fighting for equal rights for all regardless of ethnicity, appearance, sexuality or gender identity.

Some people argue that in light of the progress made for women's rights, feminism is no longer relevant. Unfortunately, we do not yet have social, political or economic equality of the sexes. Progress does not mean the fight is over; rather, it should be an inspiration to fight harder than before to achieve equality of living for all. The different phases of feminism are defined as waves, which are explained in more detail in the following pages.

What has feminism got to do with vaginas? The representation and treatment of the vagina is a key battleground for feminists across the world. Sexual health and liberty of sexuality for vagina-owners is crucial for achieving true equality and, as such, narratives around the vagina have formed an essential part of feminist discourse across each of its incarnations.

FIRST-WAVE FEMINISM

Taking place in the late nineteenth and early twentieth centuries, the first wave of feminism was fought through suffrage movements across the world. Though women had been advocating for more rights long before this wave, this was the first organized movement to achieve national and international change.

In Britain, the suffragettes and suffragists led campaigns of protest, both peaceful and active. Building on the work of writers such as Mary Wollstonecraft, the women launched hunger strikes, chained themselves to buildings and set fire to postboxes. The martyrdom of Emily Davison, who threw herself in front of the King's horse, was a turning point, as was the enormous role women played during the First World War. In 1918, landowning women were given the vote, and by 1928 this had been extended to all women over 21.

Meanwhile, the suffragettes' Stateside sisters were fighting a battle of their own. For over 100 years, American women organized and protested. For them also, the First World War was a momentous demonstration of the strength of the nation's women, and they gained the vote in 1920.

SECOND-WAVE FEMINISM

In the sixties and seventies, women were growing disillusioned with the supposed equality gained through their foremothers' struggles. Though they had the vote, women still suffered. Spurred on by the victories of their mothers before them, they began to demand change.

Unlike their first-wave sisters, second-wave feminists sought to understand the roots of oppression, with books such as Kate Millet's *Sexual Politics* and speakers including Gloria Steinem and Angela Davis greatly influencing women both in the US and across the pond in Great Britain.

The challenges of philosophical questions about gender, race and sexuality began to fracture the movement, and it splintered into subgroups. Liberal feminists focused on palpable legal change. Radical feminists didn't feel that was enough – they wanted large-scale societal change, to restructure the world in a way that redressed its balance.

Much like the first wave before it, second-wave feminism was dominated by white voices, and frequently sidelined the dual oppression of sexism and racism, erasing the experiences and voices of women of colour in the process. There was still a long way to go.

THIRD-WAVE FEMINISM

The 1990s brought us more than Tamagotchis and the Spice Girls: it heralded the dawn of third-wave feminism. This was driven by the daughters of the second wave: they'd grown up with an awareness of the inequalities still prevalent in society, and the inspiration to challenge them.

Third-wave feminists sought to subvert what they'd been taught about identity, redefining concepts of sexuality and gender. Beauty, too, was up for debate, with Naomi Wolf's *The Beauty Myth* revealing the ways Western, capitalist-driven conceptions of "beauty" were used as a tool of oppression.

Women began to claim their place in culture. The Riot Grrls punk movement took hold, and the Guerrilla Girls began to shake things up in the art scene, while singers like Mariah Carey, Whitney Houston and Mary J. Blige became power icons as the world had never seen them before, redefining and reclaiming the word "diva".

Girl power took over the mainstream, as TV, cinema and music all tried to appeal to an audience of women who demanded content that represented the new-found freedoms they were enjoying in the workplace and the bedroom.

FOURTH-WAVE FEMINISM

Since 2012, a fourth wave of feminism has begun to emerge. No longer content with the peppy "girl power" slogans of the nineties, fourth-wave feminism strives to right wrongs, expose oppressors and demand justice.

The "Me Too" movement was launched in 2006 by activist Tarana Burke, who wanted to promote empowerment through empathy for women who had survived sexual abuse. The movement gained momentum on an unprecedented scale when, in 2015, accusations against Hollywood producer Harvey Weinstein came to light, exposing years of sexual abuse within the movie industry. Across the world, women came together to share their stories with #MeToo, and demand justice for victims. During the first 24 hours of the hashtag being shared on Facebook in 2017, it had been used in 12 million posts. Finally, companies and individuals were forced to be accountable for years of abuse women had previously had to suffer in silence.

Fourth-wave feminism is developing every day and is far from perfect. Still not intersectional enough, campaigns need to do more to include and be led by the voices of women of colour and the LGBT community.

WHERE DO WE GO FROM HERE?

The fight for vagina-owners' rights is far from over. Oppression across the world is still rife. But how can you aid the cause in your day-to-day life?

Endeavour to educate yourself wherever you can on the struggles of others, especially if you are a straight, white ciswoman. Though you face discrimination based on your identity, you're also privy to great power on account of your race, gender and sexuality. Harness those privileges for good, by reading about what makes a good ally and embarking on a process of continual self-improvement.

Get involved! There are campaigns for issues affecting women across the globe happening right now – period poverty, domestic abuse, genital mutilation and transphobia are just some of the issues affecting our community, and the good news is, it's easy to play your part. Write to your politician, sign petitions, donate where you can and get out on the streets to march with your sisters and demand change.

Remember that your ancestors fought for your right to vote. Use it. It's your most powerful weapon against oppression.

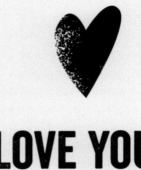

LOVE YOUR VAGINA

Having made it this far, you are hopefully reflecting on your own vagina as the miraculous organ it is – capable and strong, beautiful, unique and able to provide immense pleasure. Still struggling? This is the chapter for you. Read on to feel closer to the you between your thighs.

REMOVING PUBIC HAIR MAKES THE VAGINA CLEANER

In a 2016 survey, most women questioned claimed that they removed pubic hair in order to maintain hygiene, but there's no evidence that a hairless vagina is a cleaner vagina. In fact, removing your pubic hair can leave you more exposed to contracting STIs. This is because the process of hair removal causes micro-trauma to the pubic region, offering more portals of entry for bacteria and infection.

A full bush of pubic hair offers a barrier between the vagina and dirt or infection and so is actually the safest way to style your vagina. If you choose to remove hair, be sure to follow the advice that accompanies your chosen method, particularly gently exfoliating the area where hair has been removed to avoid painful ingrowns.

Whatever look you prefer – all-off Hollywood style, short and stubbly or shaped into a lightning bolt – what's important is making a choice that you're comfortable with and leaves you feeling sexy and confident.

THE MAGIC OF THE VAGINA

If you haven't yet learned to love your vagina, you can take comfort in the fact that it definitely loves itself! Vaginas are masters in self-care.

When your body goes through puberty, the vagina becomes home to a whole colony of healthy bacteria, which produce lactic acid. The acidity that these bacteria create in the vagina protects it from infections. This is also the reason that over time, you may notice the gusset of your underwear becomes lighter – your discharge has literally bleached the fabric.

The vaginal eco-system is very finely balanced. Together with discharge, this complex system cleans the vagina all on its own, without a need for any work from the vagina-owner.

With such a delicate cleaning system, however, comes the risk of disruption. Douches, cleaning the vagina with soaps, deodorants, scented sanitary products, or procedures aimed to "cleanse" the vagina such as "vaginal steaming" (thank Gwyneth Paltrow's Goop for that gem) can all throw this balance off and lead to serious discomfort, or even infection.

To thank your vagina for its miraculous cleaning service, simply use a plain, unscented soap around the outer vulva area each time you shower. Only ever have contact with the outside skin, never inside the lips or over the vagina itself. Resist the call of products that lay claim to making your down-there smell like roses – vaginas aren't meant to smell of anything but vagina, and anything that claims otherwise is an infection waiting to happen.

> To further protect your vagina, wear cotton underwear. Cotton is both breathable and absorbent, which will help to prevent uncomfortable yeast infections. Going commando at night also gives your vagina a chance to breathe and recover from a day in pantie prison.

COMMON VAGINA ISSUES

For all its wonders, some complications can make life with your vagina difficult. Here are some common issues, and advice on when it's time to see a doctor.

YEAST INFECTIONS

These infections, also called thrush, are caused by an overgrowth of the normally healthy bacteria, candida. This overgrowth can be caused by medication, re-wearing underwear, a weakened immune system, or sometimes no obvious cause at all. Symptoms include redness, swelling, burning, itching, pain when urinating and during sex, and thick white discharge. Head to your pharmacy for over-the-counter treatment, which usually consists of a topical cream. If symptoms persist, visit your doctor.

CYSTITIS

This common UTI presents itself as pain when urinating, an increased urge to pee, urine that is dark in colour, stomach pain or a general run-down feeling. Though these infections usually clear up after a few days, if your pain is persistent see your doctor for a course of antibiotics. The best way to treat cystitis at home is to drink plenty of water, take painkillers and use a hot-water bottle.

BACTERIAL VAGINOSIS

The most common sign of bacterial vaginosis is strong-smelling discharge that is greyish-white and/or watery in consistency. Bacterial vaginosis can leave you more prone to sexually transmitted infections and can cause complications in pregnancy, so visit your doctor for a course of antibiotics to clear up the issue.

VAGINISMUS

People with vaginismus find that their vagina tightens up, often to a painful degree, just as something – whether a penis, toy, finger or tampon – is inserted into it. This can be very distressing. Vaginismus is classified as a fear response and treatment is focused on removing this sense of fear, through exercises designed to make you more comfortable with penetration. Visit your doctor for help accessing treatment.

VAGINITIS

Soreness and swelling of the vagina are the most common signs of vaginitis, and this is often accompanied by dryness, itching, sore or cracked skin and light bleeding between periods. It's common to require a pelvic examination.

I DON'T CONSIDER MYSELF
BEAUTIFUL OR FAMOUS,
BUT MY VAGINA CERTAINLY
IS... I HAVE THE ANGELINA
JOLIE OF VAGINAS.

Amy Poehler

Remember you can always request a female doctor and ask them to stop at any point if you become uncomfortable. Treatments tend to involve creams or antibiotics.

KEEPING UP WITH THE KEGELS

Also known as pelvic floor exercises, Kegel workouts strengthen the muscles around the bladder, bottom and vagina. Though people often claim to use them to "tighten" the vagina, this isn't quite accurate, though regularly doing these exercises can make sex more enjoyable by relaxing the vaginal muscles, improving circulation to the pelvic floor and increasing wetness. Another benefit of these exercises is protection against incontinence, making them especially important for those who have given birth.

To find your pelvic floor muscles, imagine you are on the loo. Squeeze the same way you would to stop the flow of pee. When you're ready to exercise (for real benefits, you'll want to do this twice a day), get into a comfortable, relaxed position and follow these instructions.

1. Breathe in deeply. As you breathe out, gently squeeze your pelvic floor muscle.

2. Keep the muscle contracted for 5 seconds (it's okay to build up to this if it's difficult at first) and gently release with your next intake of breath.

3. Completely relax the muscle for the next cycle of breath, and then repeat the process ten times.

SMEAR TESTS

All people with a cervix aged 25–64 should attend cervical smear tests (also known as Pap tests) every three years. These tests are designed to prevent cervical cancer from developing by looking for certain kinds of HPV cells that can cause changes to the cells that make up your cervix.

Many people are apprehensive about smear tests, but with knowledge on your side, the experience doesn't have to cause anything more than slight discomfort, and you can always take an over-the-counter painkiller before your appointment to ease any tenderness. During a smear test you will be asked to lie down so that the doctor or nurse can insert a speculum into your vagina. This is a duck-bill-shaped tool that opens up slightly to allow access to your cervix. They will then use a small spatula or brush to collect cells.

The experience shouldn't be painful – alert your medical professional if it is – but it will be uncomfortable. Your doctor or nurse will send your swab off to a lab, and results are generally available within two weeks of your test. Concerned about a rushed experience? Book a double appointment, so you'll have more time to discuss the process with your doctor.

WHAT CAN GO WRONG WITH THE VAGINA?

Sometimes vagina-owners can encounter problems that go beyond the reach of antibiotics or creams. Here are some long-term issues that can affect vaginal health.

VULVODYNIA

Though the vagina looks normal, vulvodynia sufferers are subject to near constant pain that can be triggered by sitting on or touching the area. This distressing condition should be discussed with your doctor. Severe cases may require counselling, physiotherapy or surgery.

ENDOMETRIOSIS

The kind of tissue that lines the womb grows in other places too for endometriosis sufferers, including the ovaries and fallopian tubes. Though sometimes symptomless, it can cause serious problems, and often first presents as pains in the tummy and back during sex and when using the toilet. It can also cause nausea, constipation, diarrhoea, bloody urine or difficulty with becoming pregnant. See your doctor if you have these symptoms.

POLYCYSTIC OVARY SYNDROME

This condition affects how your ovaries function, resulting in high levels of "male" hormones in the body and polycystic ovaries. Symptoms include irregular or absent periods, excessive body hair growth, weight gain, acne, thinning hair and fertility issues. While there's no cure, symptoms can be treated.

EVERY VAGINA IS DIFFERENT

Every vagina on the planet is different. They are as unique as faces, and no two look truly the same. Not only are there vast differences in appearance – labia length, puffiness, colour, clitoral size – but each vagina also has its own smell, texture and discharge.

Our differences are something to celebrate! If you feel alone, or that your vagina is "abnormal", have a quick Google of photographer Laura Dodsworth, who has photographed over 100 vaginas. A BBC report in 2017 discovered that girls as young as nine were seeking surgery for their genitals because they believed they were wrong or ugly. Meanwhile, UNICEF reports that 200 million vagina-owners alive today have undergone female genital mutilation of varying kinds and severity. Speaking about her project to the BBC, Dodsworth said, "Frankly, we just need to be as we are. Yes, you can look at the photos and go 'Wow, we all look really different', but it's also about connecting with the honesty of these stories. Because if you find yourself feeling admiration, pride and inspiration for another person, it becomes easier to apply that to yourself, too."

TALK ABOUT YOUR VAGINA!

The best way to feel good about your vagina is to create an environment where you *talk* about your vagina. In opening up about your downstairs, you'll be taking the first step to eliminating the shame and taboo that prevents so many vagina-owners from seeking help and reassurance when they need it.

Studies have shown that vast swathes of women are uncomfortable with discussing their vaginal health, even with their doctors. Over half of women aged 35 and under are unable to label a diagram of their genitals correctly and more than 20 per cent say they would not attend their smear test.

Try opening up to someone you trust, whether that's discussing something that's worrying you, making a joke, or simply using the word "vagina" when you'd usually say "private parts". You'll be amazed how much impact speaking openly about your body has on your confidence. And who knows, if that means opening up to your doctor, one day it could just save your life!

CONCLUSION

Your vagina. A self-cleaning, baby-making, sexy-looking miracle between your thighs. What a wonder. Hopefully these pages have filled you with admiration for your nether regions and given you the gift of love for your vagina. However yours looks, whatever your history, know that your vagina is absolutely perfect, just as it is. And the best part? Whatever you choose to do with your vagina, from creating new life, to enjoying heart-stopping orgasms, it's nobody's business but your own.

You have ownership of the only part of the body purely created for pleasure, a magic canal that can stretch to the size of a bagel then snap back to the size of a blueberry, with a completely unique, bespoke design – it's hard to imagine feeling anything but awe for this incredible organ.

Each vagina is unique, each vagina is powerful, each vagina is capable of pleasure so intense that the French call it "the little death" (*la petite mort*). Is it any wonder our ancient ancestors worshipped the vagina as divine?

FURTHER READING

BOOKS

The Vagina Bible by Dr Jen Gunter

Vagina by Naomi Wolf

The Gynae Geek by Dr Anita Mitra

How to Have Feminist Sex by Flo Perry

Me and My Menopausal Vagina by Jane Lewis

Everything You Ever Wanted to Know About Trans by Brynn Tannehill

Yes, You Are Trans Enough by Mia Violet

WEBSITES

www.vaginamuseum.co.uk

www.bbc.co.uk/news/resources/idt-sh/Why_I_
Photographed_100_Vulvas

www.helloclue.com/articles

www.greatwallofvagina.co.uk

INSTAGRAM

@thegreatwallofvagina

@thevaginabible

@thevaginablog

@thevulvagallery

@vagina_museum

@mermaidsgender

Have you enjoyed this book? If so, find us on
Facebook at **Summersdale Publishers**, on
Twitter at **@Summersdale** and on Instagram at
@summersdalebooks and get in touch.
We'd love to hear from you!

www.summersdale.com

IMAGE CREDITS

p.37 © Julia Sanders/Shutterstock.com
p.41 © Sonias drawings/Shutterstock.com